COPING *with* CARE
of a LOVED ONE
ON THE DEMENTIA ROAD

D1722708

BARBARA RUSH-HOWARD

COPING *with* CARE *of a* LOVED ONE ON THE DEMENTIA ROAD

XULON PRESS

Xulon Press
2301 Lucien Way #415
Maitland, FL 32751
407.339.4217
www.xulonpress.com

Paperback ISBN-13: 978-1-6628-5962-5
Ebook ISBN-13: 978-1-6628-5963-2

Table of Contents

Introduction

THIS LITTLE BOOK captures my personal experience in caring for a loved one diagnosed with dementia, my husband James Howard Jr. The discovery was made after twenty-three years of a wonderful marriage, with us looking to retirement and many more years of the same. I hope to convey a story of hope, love in action, resources and support, and helpful counsel and hints, as well as ways to regenerate so neither the caregiver or loved one suffers in the things needed to live life well and fulfilled.

It is my prayer that this book will be of help to caregiver and spouse or family member with dementia. I want you to know that you are not alone on this journey. Somewhere, somehow, someone is experiencing the same kinds of issues in dealing with their loved one as well, and each of us can support one another.

I recommend you reflect on these things I have listed below as you read the remainder of what I have endeavored to present for your help, encouragement, and strength.

- Pray. God is listening and will help. He will give you peace and guidance and understanding, as well as be a light on your path to see the things you need and a joy to show and be the love your loved one requires.
- Don't panic or get frustrated as you move to wrap your mind around what you may be concerned about is ahead. This is the task that was presented to me.
- Don't be ashamed to reach out to your church, family members, and friends, as well as those who have experienced what you are facing.

- Research and make plans to utilize outside services, including, and not limited to, your family physician and community programs in your area. If your loved one has served in the military, be sure to engage the Veteran's Administration and Social Security or Medicaid or Medicare for any literature or guidance or social workers.

- Don't be overwhelmed by what you may see at first as "financial" impacts. There may not be much help out there for financial advice, so the support of family and friends is important, unless there are already long-term care remedies in place.

- Emotional support is critical to maintaining perspective of the caregiver mission and dementia patient needs. Physical wellbeing is an important factor for both too.

- It is very important to let go of hate, grudges, and bitterness and forgive. It is not the caregiver in battle against the patient. You will find a kind of peace that helps us to go on with our life and be fulfilled in it.

- Pray. God is listening and will help.

Life has many challenges, and some are completely unexpected, as with a loved one having dementia. However, God is present always with us to show brand new mercies, give us the wisdom and strength to overcome, provide joyful visions of better possibilities, and help us to live rewarding lives despite the challenges—even dementia. God gives us the opportunity to make choices. I thank God I chose to stand with my loved one when dementia Hit.

Acknowledgements

MY FIRST AND foremost acknowledgement is to my Lord and Savior Jesus Christ. I am so grateful to God, Who gave me the vision, inspiration, wisdom, and the ability, along with a few good people, needed to help tell my story.

TO GOD BE THE GLORY

The reason I decided to tell my story is I believe I have something positive to contribute that would reflect acts of care and concern for your loved ones when a medical or mental crisis arises. I pray that my story will be of some help to the readers.

My desire for writing this is for self-gratification and not about making money. I always thought that I had potential to reach out with a short story of knowledge to help others, and by doing this, it made sense for me to put my efforts into making it happen.

The good news is that God is God. He is capable of handling what we can't and also what is impossible for us but is possible for God to handle.

Below, I would like to acknowledge the people who I know have helped and would like them to be recognized in print.

To my pastor the Honorable Elder Abe Elliott Jr. and my entire church family, Elliott Chapel Free Will Baptist Church, for all prayers, calls, and concerns. I thank you for your love and support.

To my husband's daughter, Trenita Howard, son, James Howard, and daughter-in-law, Anika Howard, for all the love, concern, and outstanding support for which I am so grateful.

To John M. Ray, MD, his primary physician, for his care and concern, as well as friendship and kindness, during this time of need. I am forever grateful.

To my son, David D. Rush, who stuck by my side with helping with the personal care and ran errands when needed, but most of all, for spending time with him on most Sundays to allow me to attend church services as often as he could. Thank you for always being there for me.

To my sister, Connie L. Martin, thank you for your love, strong support and commitment, and for all you do to help ease my burden. I want you to know I love you and thank you for the bottom of my heart.

To my brother, Charles Martin, and his wife, Sandra Martin. The best brother and sister you could ask for. Thank you for your love and great support.

To Darin Martin, my nephew. I thank you for all the prayers, support, and confidence in me that helped me to keep going. I thank God for what you bring to my life.

To my dear friend Nadine Berry. Without her love, strong support, and assistance, I could have not gotten my manuscript done. I am so grateful.

To Orga Price for his input and expertise in helping me with the finishing touches of my manuscript.

To my dear friends Elder Mattie Curry, Minister Ann V. Hurley, and Sister Regina Ray for spiritual support encouragement and comforting when my spirit was low. Thank you.

To Aunt Ruth, cousins Gladys, Theresa, Tiara, the Jackson family and the McQueen family, and all other family and friends in Cheraw, South Carolina.

To Dr. Cedric Wooten (aka as Dr. Woo) for the feedback, guidance, help, and support I needed to finish writing this book. I am forever grateful.

To my dear friend Cheryle T. Ricks for encouragement and support, connecting me to a great publishing company with extraordinary staff.

If I didn't acknowledge you personally, please forgive me; however, if you expressed concern, I am truly thankful for your support and concern and prayers.

Thanks again for you love, prayers, and concern, and above all, God bless and keep you all, my family and friends.

The Big Hit Dementia

MY HUSBAND WAS diagnosed with dementia in 2015. It came on him slow and gradual and very unnoticeable at first. I will say, he had a good sense of humor and at times would play it off in the beginning. This condition went on for over a year or so. Then things changed with him. I noticed that he started misplacing things of importance like his jewelry, keys, mail, and appointment dates. The next major sign was that he began to feel uncomfortable driving, which I know now, in hindsight, was impacted by his uncertainty, due to the fact that he was losing his ability of recall from one destination to the other. Soon after, he suddenly stopped driving all together without being told to do so.

At that time, I realized he was in trouble, which, of course, was very hard for me. Now the table was turned for me to make all decisions and accept all the responsibility of running the household along with more engaged and intimate providing of care for him.

Dementia is a chronic or persistent disorder of the mental process which goes through seven stages until death. As this disease progresses, there will be noticeable changes in the patient as well. Dementia can be caused by many factors as well. For example, besides brain disease or injury, chronic high blood pressure, known as hypertension, can cause dementia and disposition by genetic background in the family. Noticeable changes from dementia that are observable are memory loss issues, personality changes, and impaired reasoning, as well as repeating in conversation the same memory of the past over and over. These examples advance in complexity until in the final stages: not knowing or recognizing who your loved one is, with episodes of your loved one not talking at all or reverting to a child. A difficult and stressful time to lose that connection with someone so dear and near to you.

The first signs are subtle and can be easily missed. Of course, the subtlety coupled with denial and disbelief and associated anxiety can make it difficult to accept. However there is medications that can be prescribed by the doctor, that can ease symptoms for a while, or slow down the progression. Medication does not cure the disease but they do somehow improve the quality of life and help prolong the independence in some people.

The fact is that the spouse or the caregiver must come to grips, that this will be on going and become a more difficult process due to the overall deterioration of your loved one.

The time will come when your love one will have no control of bodily functions such as dressing, undressing, using the toilet, bathing, shaving and other personal hygiene needs. They may have a decrease in appetite, and mobility due to age.

Once you have accepted what is happening, it is important that you engage and be motivated to begin to formulate a strategy of how you are going to deal with the condition your loved one and you are facing. Don't rest in disbelief, convincing yourself and responding as though he/she know what they are doing or saying. Also, don't hide in fear or be incapacitated, but move to increase your knowledge and vision with identifying helpful resources that will guide you through this process. Certain tasks whether small or large your loved one will not be cable of doing at some point and will not become yours. You may find yourself becoming very frustrated, but don't give up. Allow them to continue to do what they can do for themselves even if it takes more time for them to get the task done. Align yourself with doctors who have had dementia patients or can recommend another advocate who can help you with this. Remember, every day will be different, where some days are good and other days are just downright hard.

Below is a list that I have come up with for coping with my spouse:

- Connect to the almighty God for strength along with getting deeply rooted in spirt and prayer. By doing this, it will give you the faith in moving through each issue with confidence with your loved one.
- By prayer, you will get the peace of God that comes with patience and compassion. The most important thing to remember is that he/she must become your very best friend.

Getting to this level is going to take a lot of time and patience, which could take months or even years before it all settles in. Don't beat yourself up; just take it one day at a time.

Next are a few pointers on what you need to do for yourself to keep yourself ready for the task in front of you:

- Strength – Consider your physical health and well-being.
- Peace – That, only God can provide.
- Patience – To endure and maintain the struggle.
- Compassion – from the love of God to operate in a loving and kind matter.

In other words, you will be fighting the right fight in the right way to be able to succeed in finding a sense of accomplishment in how you are handling what you are facing on this long journey on the dementia Road.

Nutrition and Personal Supplies

DIET PROBABLY WOULD not normally be a considered as a factor that can help in the care of a loved one for a disease that affects the brain. However, it is very important to plan the diet, as it can affect your loved one with dementia and possibly cause problems, such as diarrhea or vomiting. Because dementia affects the normal habits of a person, even to the point of not doing essential things such as drinking water regularly or taking prescriptions for chronic illnesses, it is important to be sensitive to diet practices to not needlessly impact your loved one in negative ways as well as increase associated work for yourself in recovery.

Make diet plans and note in a booklet any discovered sensitivities for them or habits that you need to incorporate regarding food combinations in meals, drinks, and snacks. You may need to be creative in your tracking and set reminders. Use whatever tools you are comfortable with which work for you. An example is using a cell phone to keep your information or a notebook and catalog your information with added alarms or timers to ensure you stay on schedule and information is handy for review and update. Sticky note reminders can be a temporary, quick way to help create routines and highlights for further consideration. Your tracking and reminders can help avoid foods and drinks that may cause diarrhea or vomiting for your loved one. The trackers and reminders with timers may help you to encourage your loved one to drink water on a timely, regular basis to prevent dehydration and, possibly, a urinary tract infection (UTI). UTIs are one of the biggest issues for a dementia patient, as the illness is subtle, and signs may not be communicated by patient or readily considered by caregiver for treatment. They can require hospitalization for UTIs when left untreated and infect the bloodstream and become life threatening.

As you plan for sensitivities to diet, don't neglect planning for recovery as well. Make a list of all the supplies you will need and always have them handy, such as latex gloves, Kleenex, soap, sanitizer, disinfectant, and whatever else the patient might need.

Safe Proofing Your Home

As conscientiously, purposefully, and lovingly preparation is done for a new child coming into the home to ensure no things or places in the home put a child in harm's way, you will need to adult-proof your home, making sure that everything has been locked down and is secure. Start making your lists of areas and things that need to be addressed or possibly included before incidents occur. Update that list as the changes are seen in habits new and old that impact the safety of your loved one. Your list of considered protections will support thoughtful, needed, and impactful adjustments you make in your home to safeguard your loved one. Some things to get your thoughts centered on possible changes needed are:

1. Keeping medications in pill trackers and, possibly, in unreachable or locked areas

2. Keeping chemical products in unreachable or locked areas

3. Keeping weapons in unreachable or locked areas

4. Keeping matches, lighters, and flammable products in unreachable or locked areas

5. Prevent falls in the tub/shower with a non-skid pad in place.

6. Keeping external doors locked with key not in plain sight for convenient use; a door lock may be added to external doors so key is required for exit.

7. Alarmed external doors may be an alternative consideration to keyless lock for exit or increased security.

8. Security cameras installed, internal and external, to support vision and track habits

9. Adult-proof kitchen to prevent unsupervised or undesired cooking; stove turned on but not lit for gas; hot eyes ignored, hot things, such as coffee or things cooked, not recognized.

Secure the kitchen area and all areas of the home in general. Be safe and not sorry. Be diligent in your review of the home dangers, as the ones listed above may not be the only items and places you need to consider in order to keep your loved one and those in your home safe.

Maintaining a Cheerful Patient

YOUR LOVED ONE with dementia does not require constant quiet or isolation. Enjoy the time with your loved one even though things are not the same. There will be moments of clarity and other times, seemingly, your loved one may be nonresponsive. Yet, it is very helpful to keep the patient routinely occupied to promote feeling useful. Emotions are still at work in your loved one though not always expressed, and attendance to them is important to the wellbeing for a healthy response. Remember, sharpening your sensitivities to the patient's awareness can lead to some very gratifying moments for patient and caregiver. Engaging your loved one in chores can promote good feelings of self-worth and lessen feelings of being burdensome or helpless. Find the projects that can be accomplished like folding clothes or other things your loved one engages in without resistance. It is very important that you allow them to do the things they can do for themselves for as long as they can do the project. Projects should not be time constrained and be supported with compliments for encouragement and emphasis that performing the project matters and their support is appreciated. By doing this, it allows them to still maintain purpose despite what they are going through. It is critical you maintain the perspective that you are not the only one going through the change. Your loved one is challenged as well and can be as frustrated as you trying to work it out in their mind too. Imagine them saying to themselves, "What is going on with me?" and saying, "I was able to do this and now I can't figure out what I am doing." You are not alone, as there is support for you, and they are not alone as you demonstrate your love in caring for them.

Some things you can incorporate into routines that help are a) engaging them in physical exercise like walking to the mailbox daily b) putting out the trash, or c) just sweeping the floor. You may incorporate hobbies, perhaps scaled back versions, that your loved one enjoyed, such as gardening, listening to their favorite music in their favorite place, or taking a short drive in the car. You will surely be surprised how doing little chores can help make a person cheerful, and experiencing elements of things and places that were frequent a part of their life can inspire them to happier levels.

Legal Documents that You Need to Have in Order to Make Decisions for Your Loved One

As you can expect, the legal matters that have to be addressed are apart from the personal care of your loved one. However, legal framework must be in place for you to support your loved one in decisions regarding their health, personal business matters, where care is rendered, who care is rendered by, and their estate. The proper legal authority to authorize care and business transactions as needed is a legal matter. This will include legal identification of a trusted, reliable alternate in case you cannot fulfill your responsibility in the entity of an institution or person. The legal framework needs to occur early in the dementia stages for ease and smooth execution with the participation of your loved one to sign off on authority given and any alternate persons or paths recommended for care. Otherwise, securing the legal framework needed may be unattainable and left to federal or state institutional remedies with you on the sideline and, perhaps, no straight path to participate without another legal pursuit of declaration.

It is very important that you obtain all the necessary legal documents that will put you in the position to handle and make the decisions in the care of loved one. To do this, you must have a dual power of attorney (POA) and a health care proxy (HCP). To accomplish securing these documents through the legal system, your loved one must be in a legally defined "reasonable state of mind" and in agreement and able to sign the paperwork that must also be notarized by a notary with active certificate. Additional things to accomplish for during business transactions using funds your loved one has: Make sure that your name is on your loved one's savings and checking account and you are the beneficiary of any other legal documents in their possession (insurance policies, bonds, stocks, money market accounts, pensions, 401K or IRA plans, and real estate that is in their name only). By having these documents in order and in place, you will have the authority to be their voice when they have no voice. All of these documents can be drafted by your family attorney at a cost which, typically, is not very costly but necessary. The attorney may have additional recommendations for paperwork based on federal, state, or local guidelines.

The Other Person Who Needs to Be Maintained

YOU ARE THE other person who needs to be cared for to make caring for a loved one with dementia successful. There are many things to accomplish, and being organized and prepared will help tremendously, but you must take care of yourself. Set aside time for yourself to do what is needed for YOU. Main recommendations include:

- Take regular breaks away/eat healthy.
- Be sure that your needs are included in your daily routine.
- Take naps during the day whenever possible so you are at your best and alert.

- Get a good night of rest each night (safeguarding and securing home will help).
- Heighten your sensitivities to be aware of changes in your loved one and be mindful you are not in a fight with your loved one to use wisdom to overcome obstacles and dilute frustration.

Be open with supportive family and friends and talk about how you are feeling and dealing emotionally handling caregiver issues. Having conversations with family members and friends who have the time and want to be in your corner for support is very necessary as well.

Everyone's situation in caring for a loved one with dementia may have difference, especially driven by what stage of dementia the patient is in. There are times when thoughts will come to them so clearly and that the mind is clearer than a bell. It's hard to say, but you need to remember it's mostly a temporary situation and enjoy it and be inspired by it, even in its brevity.

Try to manage your time, energy, and emotions to support maneuvering through situations when they come your way. There is no greater assurance for you or your loved one than knowing God is with you and you can lean on Him and talk to Him for comfort and strength. Again, remember to keep your personal relationship with God. You will have your guardian angels of grace and mercy there for protection of yourself and your loved one. Keep these words in your mind: "With God's help everything is possible."

Make a Priority List of Issues that You Deal with When it Comes to Mind on How to Deal with an Issue

EVERY ISSUE IS an issue, but every issue has its own priority based on impact to your loved one's wellbeing and yours too. One of the items identified to include on your list of things to be accomplished is that "you must maintain a strong position of control and maintain a very authoritative attitude." Always speak clearly and with a calm voice when you are trying to get the patient to do any tasks. Using this technique with the patient will most times get the patient to do what is being asked of them to do. Be sure to keep your frustration level away from the conclusion that they want to be stubborn and very uncooperative at times to diffuse your frustration level. Both you and your loved one are in a foreign land called "dementia" and have to learn the language on the job. I encourage you to learn to let things go and seek alternatives to battling, including even to wait till another day to try a different approach. If you respond too quickly to every little thing when you could have stepped back and approached it a different way to achieve the result you wanted, you could push yourself toward burnout. You should pause and ask yourself certain questions like "Is it worth how I am feeling now, emotionally drained, and still nothing has been accomplished?" Keep in mind you are not dealing with the normal habits of the person you remember any longer but dealing with a loved one who is only following what their mind is telling them to do. With this approach, you will keep centered and calm and prevent blood pressure from rising.

Facing the Trials Head On

ALL I HAVE communicated in this short help book on caring for a loved one with dementia is not necessarily fully descriptive of your journey. Oh yes, there may be many experiences on your journey that don't align to my witness here. Don't be afraid, but let love guide you to handle challenges head on. Issues may come without warning and the surprise is not just to you but also your loved one who has no desire to add to your workload of caregiving to them. Maintain your posture of love and keep your head high, remembering all that your loved one means to you and how much you mean to them and are depended on and trusted in. Have an umbrella of support if you need to get out of the rain to dry off and strategize on your approaches to issues. Your loved one is worth the challenges you overcome and changes you endure as your love energizes and God gives you wisdom on your response to each issue and next course of action. Continue to move forward while leaning on God for your strength and your encouragement, remembering both you and your loved one win. God will provide everything you need, and when you have completed your path, you can say JOB WELL DONE, my love was demonstrated and certified.

To conclude, I say remember you are not alone on the path that is before you. Stay calm, prayerful, having that personal relationship with God is very essential when storms come and go. To make the right decisions you must be led by the spirit of God. God will always guide us and he will show up in ways we never think. You can't confide in just anyone when God sent to you the right person to help you will know. When God is in the equation you will experience so much more about who he is and how much he loves, and strengthens all of us that trust and believe in his love, his word and his everlasting promises. That has been my strong hold as I go through this difficult journey at this time. Through it all my life is blessed and good. Knowing that God is our only hope when have these feelings of throwing your hands up and walking away. Don't doubt him and his power of unburdening you he is always there watching and listening. He will direct your thoughts and you will remain steady and in control of uncertain situations that you are going through at that time.

Reach out to those family members and friends that God has placed in your life along with the resources available to you with the confidence and inner peace that you and your loved one will be well through the process. Know that the almighty God is your primary source and others are orchestrated by him, for he is the only one that can really help you.

I am just an ordinary person who found myself on a extraordinary journey. In sharing my story, it is my hope that it helps bring into your vision the inspiration, professional and all other support and resources necessary in going through the stages along with them on the dementia path.

I have to say, finally we can begin to fear less and make fewer wrong mistakes by embracing better ways we can care for our loved ones having dementia.

Know that there is power in allowing yourself to make known and heard in owning our unique story in using your real voice.

Know that everyday life can be difficult at times, as we struggle to complete our task.

But There is Jesus!!!

About the Author:
Barbara Rush-Howard

I WAS BORN in Rockville, Maryland to Charles R. Martin and Mary Margaret Martin.

My parents moved to Washington, D.C. when I was very young. I attended the D.C. Public School system and graduated from M.M. Washington Vocational High in 1964. I was married thereafter and gave birth to a son, David D. Rush. In 1966, I started my work career with the federal government where I worked in various positions. Shortly afterward, my marriage ended, and I became a single mom and continued to work and take care of my son. Some years later, I met James Howard Jr., and we got married.

After thirty years of government service, I retired my position as a program analyst. Since my husband I were both retired, we decided to move to North Carolina where we are still living at this time of writing of this book.

I have always seen myself as a passionate private person. I try to focus on the good things in life. My personal spiritual search has reached new heights during the health experience with my husband. It is my intent to share God's love with others and anyone else who cares to use my personal experiences as an inspiration to the reader.

It is my feeling that the best cure for dementia is living and loving the patient with everything that you have inside of you.

Again, I want to Thank God for everything especially for his love for my caring for my husband on the Dementia Road.

List of Noticeable Challenges and Effects of the Changes in the Characteristics of Your Loved One Over a Period of Time When Onset Dementia Is Coming on:

- memory loss that disrupts daily life and routine
- challenges in planning and solving problems
- difficulty completing familiar tasks
- trouble understanding visual images and, in particular, knowing one person from another and also what their relationship is with them
- confusion with times and places
- problem with speech and writing
- misplacing items
- decreased or poor judgement in accomplishing tasks
- withdrawal from simple task and social activities

- mood changes in the personality; in particular, becoming stubborn or will not cooperate
- unsteady when walking and wandering because they have forgotten where they are
- hallucinating and confusion along with sleep disorder
- One of the biggest challenges is the personal care of the patient, regarding bathing, brushing teeth, shaving, dressing, and keeping them active in making this happen.

HELFUL RESOURCES
DEMENTIA CHARITY
24/7 HELPLINE 800-272-3900

Get involved with your local chapter
in your area

Get the facts needed from the research institutes below:

NIH (National Institute of Health)
Bethesda, MD

Johns Hopkins University
Baltimore, MD 877-552-2306

Dementia Society of American/Charity
Organizations
Doylestown, PA 949-652-7301

University of North Carolina (UNC)
Department of Neurology Chapel Hill
919-966-7233

Duke Neurology Research Center
Located Raleigh, NC and Durham, NC

Patient and community resources/care-givers organizations available and check your local area.

King James Version of Bible Verses For Strength and Encouragement

Listed is just a few sources of Bible verses to meditate on that will inspire you to find strength, courage and confidence needed to get through the toughest problems life throws at you.

John	16: 33
Isaiah	41: 10, 41: 13
Philippians	2: 3-4, 4: 6-7
Joshua	1: 9
Romans	8: 15:13, 8:28
Matthew	6: 31-34
Proverbs	3: 5-6
2 Corinthians	7: 14
1 Peter	5: 6-7
Psalms	34: 4-5, 34: 8, 94: 18-19, 121: 1-2
Revelation	21: 4

I, pray that these bible verses help you and remind you of the hope we have in OUR LORD AND SAVIOR JESUS CHRIST.

AMEN

CPSIA information can be obtained
at www.ICGtesting.com
Printed in the USA
BVHW081428121122
651756BV00010B/1148

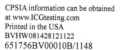

9 781662 859625